# WALKING THROUGH
# ANXIETY AND DEPRESSION

# Walking Through Anxiety and Depression

LISA LAWRENCE

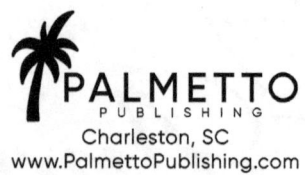

Charleston, SC
www.PalmettoPublishing.com

*Walking through Anxiety and Depression*
Copyright © 2023 by Lisa Lawrence

All rights reserved
No portion of this book may be reproduced, stored in a retrieval system, or transmitted in any form by any means–electronic, mechanical, photocopy, recording, or other–except for brief quotations in printed reviews, without prior permission of the author.

First Edition

Paperback ISBN: 979-8-8229-2449-9

*I dedicate this book to my oldest son, Casey. He is the one who prodded me to write. He came over with a journal and two brand-new ink pens. He believed in me, which in turn caused me to believe in myself. So I began to write.*

My story begins somewhere. With everything I've been through in my life, it's hard (very hard) to find that beginning. I have bipolar disorder. Not only that, but I have suffered with anxiety and depression.

First off, let me point out that I am not a doctor. I am just a regular person like the rest of us. The difference is that I have owned my mental illness. I have accepted it, and I have dealt with it for many years.

My family has been through hell and back because of me. Somewhere, however, in the midst of things, I have tried to learn to forgive myself because it wasn't me—it was the illness.

I am happy to say that I haven't had any problems for thirteen years. Let me rephrase that. I haven't been erratic. I have and still deal with anxiety.

My anxiety comes from a place of feeling overwhelmed. Perhaps like there is more for me to do than I can handle. Stress, oh that enemy word, s-t-r-e-s-s! Do you know how bad stress affects us? Our children want to grow up so fast. What are they racing for? A grown-up world that is full of stress and maybe even some forms of mental deficiencies.

When I was a little girl, I don't remember experiencing any stress, besides just trying really hard to behave myself so that I didn't get a spanking.

I remember wanting to grow up so fast to be on my own. At age fifteen, I was ready to get married and start having babies, have my own family. I did get married at eighteen and had my first baby at age twenty-one.

As you continue to read this book, you will find that *love* is the theme. I was always a love child. I needed love so bad. The words "I love you" were never spoken in my home, to nobody and by nobody. There was no show of affection. Nobody touched or hugged. We all just kind of walked around each other. When I say "we all," I am speaking of my mother and father and myself. I was an only child.

I suppose I never knew the absence of love until I started going over to my friend's house. They always said, "I love you," and kissed and hugged each other. The awareness of that caused me to start doubting that my mom and dad loved me.

I was in desperate need of love and affection. So what did I do? I went looking for love in a boyfriend. As I write this, I can't tell you how important it is to show your kids love and affection, and please don't forget to touch them.

It wasn't until I was grown that I started realizing that I really was loved by my parents. You know we can do everything that we think is right at the moment with raising our kids, and somewhere in the midst of time, it will never have been good enough. My parents did their best. I have come to realize that as an adult.

So if we're talking about depression, I would say I had my fair share as a teenager and young adult. I think my depression came from focusing on the negative aspects of my life, instead of the positive. I can't remember ever being that thankful and grateful for my blessings. Thank God I was raised by two parents who really did love me. We may have been "some" poor, but we always had good food to eat because my dad raised a garden every year. I always loved my veggies as a child.

Today I am pretty much free of major depression, and I am happy. I am, however, deeply thankful to God for all I am and all I have. I try very hard not to take too much for granted.

I might not have depression at this point in my life, but, boy, do I deal with a lot of anxiety. I stay as nervous as a long-tailed cat in a room full of rocking chairs. Yes, I am on medication for anxiety. When I was a young adult, I didn't believe in or take medication. I wouldn't even take an aspirin. I was hard-core. I gave birth to my babies naturally. I have since then changed, and I now believe that God has given us the meds to help. Help is the greatest thing. I believe you are reading this book because you want to help yourself. Reading about someone else's struggles helps us to realize we are not alone with our problems. Anxiety and depression are *big* problems because they can consume our very existence. Any kind of mental health disorder can really do you in. For me, you can add bipolar disorder.

Even with all the education we have today about mental health disorder, there is still a big stigma that goes along with it. I have lost dear friends in the past because they were *afraid* of me. Today this still hurts me. I could not help anything about who I was. Because I found a good medicine and I quit drinking alcohol, I am a better me today. Guess what my doctor told me. He said, "Lisa, you cannot have any stress in your life." After he said that, I thought to myself, "Yeah right." How can you live in such a stressful world, without any stress? The answer is you can't! I have a wonderful husband who has walked with me for thirteen years. He takes care of mostly everything. He does this to keep the stress off of me. I am forever grateful to him and forever grateful to God for sending him my way.

No, stress and anxiety will never go away. It's been my experience that even though my bipolar disorder is managed, I still have it. I will never be free from it until I am free from this body and inherit a glorious new body. As you continue to read on, you will come to learn that I have a strong—yes, very strong—faith in God and with God. God lives and breathes through me. I am not a religionist; however, I am not one to go to church on Sunday and then point the finger at everyone else throughout the week. I believe that through some of my toughest times, for fifty-six years, God has helped me through. Without God I know I would not be here today. My happiness comes through him and the antidepression meds that God gave those smart people to invent. Even though I do not suffer from depression now, I can still remember what it felt like when I did. Depression for me was physically crippling. I was zapped. No energy. You can't function. You just want to sleep. That was my experience. Like I said, I take an antidepressant, and it works great. If you are struggling with depression, find yourself a good psychiatrist. There is help all around us, so just reach out and grab it.

After you've found a good doctor, start doctoring your own self. Whatever your circumstance, say to yourself, "It can always get worse, or be worse." Start seeing your glass as half full instead of half empty. Cry out to God and let God help you. And by all means, *hang in there,* until things or your mind gets better. Speaking of our mind, it holds the key to our wellness. A mind full of trash leads to anxiety and depression. Try to get rid of the trash. Try to fill your mind with good, positive thoughts. Dream of winning the lottery and then start buying tickets. When you fill your head with good thoughts, there is no room for the bad. This is hard to do, but practice makes perfect. Go through the motion in your head as if you had all the money you could spend. Some may think this sounds crazy, but dreaming is or should be part of our very existence. This puts us into a meditative state. When you're making plans to be blessed, you just might get blessed. Do away with all those negative thoughts and worries. Dream! The sky is the limit!

It's hard to have time to work on our mental health with all the hustles and bustle of today's world. I call them distractions. These distractions take away our very peace. Peace is a medicine for good health. The more meditation you can do, the more peace you have. Even God tells us in the Bible to be calm as a dove. Lord, give me the serenity to accept the things I cannot change. There are so many things that we worry about that we just cannot change. Worrying about it is a waste of time, and it adds stress *unto* you. That's when you need to step back and count your blessings. My daddy used to tell me, "Why be stressed when you're so blessed?" Sadly, there have been many stressed people I have encountered. When I ask these people to tell me something good about their life, they can't come up with one thing. These same people had a nice, warm home, a good job, and food, and the list goes on and on. Yet they themselves could not count one thing that they were thankful for. Another saying is, "Why be depressed when you're so blessed?"

I tell you, counting your blessings every single day really helps. Every morning when I get that first cup of coffee, I thank Jesus for a hot cup of coffee. Because I love coffee so much, I couldn't imagine my life without it. We live in Savannah, Georgia. When the hurricanes came through and the power was off, we would always find a way to make coffee. Isn't that funny? Something so small to be grateful for.

Still after we do all of this, counting our blessings and all, that stupid thing we call mental illness will probably be there. Feelings will always be there. We may feel up, or we may feel down. My mom and I always say, "Sometimes you're up; sometimes you're down." Just last night I was feeling a little down. But I feel much better this morning.

Let's talk about hanging on. Because things are constantly changing, so do our feelings as well. Oh, do we wish we could get up and stay up, stay feeling good. When we get down, we just have to hang on! We have to hang on because we know we aren't always going to feel this way. We will be up before long. Sometimes it may take a while. That can be the hardest part. Hanging on isn't easy but necessary to get to being up again. I think about those poor souls who take their own life. They feel as though their situation will never change. They cannot see light at the end of their tunnel. They give up. Never, ever give up. There is always light at the end of your tunnel. When you give up hope and faith, you give up everything. Hope produces joy and happiness.

Be an overcomer of mental deficiencies. Think positive! Dream of a wonderful future. When a negative thought or thoughts come into your mind, stop it and replace it with a good thought or something you are thankful for. Draw the forces of the universe unto you. I know this is true because I would get into a meditated state and dream about winning the lottery. After a couple of years, I ended up with a brand-new car and a brand-new home with no money down. I am still amazed at how this happened.

Controlling your mind and thoughts is not an easy thing to do, but practice makes perfect. You may bring your mind to something good and then your mind seems to babble away. I say babble because it does just that. We think about things that are completely wasteless. Just babbling and babbling away. Dream about something good that you want, and keep dreaming. Just watch the universe bless you with good things.

Being thankful is also a big part of being happy. It's so easy to take things for granted.

I am so blessed that I even have the ability to write these words. I am so blessed this morning to have a nice, hot cup of coffee. God only knows what I'd be like if I didn't have my coffee. People who are thankful seem to have a peace.

While you practice all these things, don't forget the professionals. Still see a doctor, and still get your medicine. These things all work together for the good of you.

Good, you know, is always fighting evil or bad. It's like me and my mama say, "Sometimes you're up; sometimes you're down," then we laugh. We make light of our deepest moments. When we're down, we say, "Well, it could always be worse." By saying that you're not making light of the bad times; you're just helping yourself get through it until you're up again. Depression usually comes when there is no *hope*. Hope is a wonderful thing, yet so many lack it. They think negative thoughts, which drain the body. My hope is in God. He has done so much for me already, and I know there is more to come. Oh, I'm not saying there might not be some bumps in the road, but with his help, I'll get through just fine. We can't help bumps. God never promised us a rose garden, or maybe he did, and we just get stuck by a thorn every now and then. We need to learn to break off and throw away these thorns. And do not leave any remnants in the skin. These remnants can still be alive and cause great infection. Thorns are like bad memories. If we continue to relive these bad memories, it will cause sickness to us. It's really amazing how many mental deficiencies we can incur onto ourselves. Reliving the past is harmful, that is if it is a bad past thought or thoughts.

Think in the present or look forward to a glorious future. Control your mind. If you are sunk so far into depression, and you can't seem to find *any* help, then just do baby steps. Go out and get yourself a great meal. When your food comes to the table, take a second and thank God for it, or take a few bites and then thank God for good taste buds.

If you are someone who does not gather joy by eating, then do like I do: dream about winning the lottery. Oh yeah, and don't forget to buy a ticket. You can't win if you don't play. Dream and let God do the rest. I am living proof that dreaming will lead to good things. Some people may say that this is a waste of time, but don't listen to them! Filling your head with good things far outdoes sitting around worrying or regretting. We bought a brand-new car. Shortly after that we bought a brand-new home with no money down. We were the first to live in it. I pulled the positive energy from the universe, and God blessed it! Try it! It works!

If you are suffering, just hold on, my dear friend. I remember not too long ago my granddaughter was brokenhearted over something.

I wrote her a long letter and gave it to her. I figured she would be apt to listen better if she read it. In that letter I told her not to worry, and that I promised. She would laugh again. I make you, my dear friend, the same promise. Guess what, my granddaughter was hot on the phone that evening laughing with one of her friends. Her problem had been solved, and she was happy again. You, my dear one, will be happy again.

Pain comes in different degrees. I think losing someone you love in death is probably the hardest. The closest person to me that I've lost is my daddy. We were close. You may think I'm crazy, but I talk to him more now than when he walked this earth. That helps me not to hurt. I don't cry over losing him because I have him all the time now. Everybody has a different belief system.

I'm the person who deals with anxiety. It seems like my plate is always overloaded, at least for me. The least little thing sends me over the top. I think a lot of my anxiety was inherited, but my mind can sometimes be my worst enemy. When I catch myself thinking negatively, I will stop dead in my tracks. If I didn't know this technique, there's no telling how bad off I would be.

Being bad off is a bad feeling. I've been there, so I know how both anxiety and depression feel. It's a weight. It's hard. It's very hard. Just remember, *hold on*. My sweet mother and I say, "Sometimes you're up, and sometimes you're down." That's just life. Life has to be lived. Whether you realize it or not, we have much more good than bad. It's just that we escalate the bad, we call in the mire, and we make the bad worse than it has to be. Having the attitude of "Well, it could always be worse" can be a blessing for us. It helps us see our glass as half full, instead of half empty.

Don't get me wrong; I think our aches and pains should be recognized by others, and we should be babied and nurtured until we are better. Love from others helps us heal. There is nothing wrong with some good chicken soup! When others are concerned about how we feel, it gives us the umph to get better. Love is one of the greatest healing agents. There is nothing wrong with babying someone when they're down. It only helps them get back up sooner. Remember to balance yourself. Love someone but don't cripple them. They have to find their own inner strength as well.

Let's talk about that word "balance." Being balanced can help us with anxiety and depression. We have to balance our thinking. Most of the time, when we are either anxious or depressed, we are having negative thoughts. Our glass is half empty instead of half full. Balance that glass out. Pour a little of God's water into your glass. Think about all the *good* things in your life. Count your blessings one by one. So many times, and so sadly, I would ask someone what they were thankful for. Their reply was that they could not produce one thing. How sad, and how sad for that poor soul. I remember one time I was venting to my sweet daughter. I was telling her everything that was going wrong with me. She simply replied, "Mama, is your glass half full or half empty?" That's what she had to say to get me back on course. Sometimes we just have to be reminded, and reminded, and reminded, over and over again. That's ok. Because we have so many distractions in life, it is very hard to remember. That's why this book will have to be read more than once. Keep it fresh in your head.

Remember, the difficult times and feelings will come. Our job is to *hold on* until they pass. Trust me—it will pass because nothing ever stays the same, and things are always changing, including your feelings. Remember my late daddy's saying, "Feelings will come, and feelings will go. What really matters is what you know." Oh boy, those feelings can really take a toll on us; it's the bad feelings I'm talking about. The doom and gloom. The doom and gloom come from doomy and gloomy thoughts. Controlling your mind and your thoughts is very difficult. Just remember, *practice makes perfect*! Just like anything else, the more you do it, the better you get at it.

Life is really worth living. We have so much more good than bad if we can just see it that way. Remember, all our blessings come from above, and one thing we can count on is God. He is always with us and will never let us down. When we get down, God *shall* always be with us to help back us up, that is if we are not bitter and angry. Please don't allow yourself to become bitter and angry. That will only take the healing process longer. Become humble. Cry instead of swear. If you are the type of person who tries to hold back the tears, *don't*. Tears are a natural release of pain. It is good to cry when you are hurting.

Speaking of hurting, I hurt when I have had anxiety and depression. It is a type of pain that none of us want to have. Many times it is not understood by others around us. Sometimes people around us may say, "Snap out of it," but anxiety, depression, or any other mental deficiency can't just be snapped out of. There have been many times when I called for professional help or just a good friend to talk to. If God has called you to be a good friend to someone who is depressed or anxious, please try to talk less and listen more. That's why God gave us two ears and one mouth. Hurting people need to be heard. They don't need to listen to your solution for them. If you are the one hurting and you don't have anyone to hear you, then I suggest you write. Write to someone you care about, and write down how you feel, then give it to them when you see them again. I'm sure they are interested enough to read it.

When you're experiencing mental deficiencies, never feel alone, because there is always someone who cares. Even if you're a person who has no family in the world, there are strangers who care. There are all kinds of programs that can help you, so just find one and start crying out for help. Everybody needs help at some time or another in their life, some more than others. Whatever you do, never, ever, ever compare yourself to anyone else. We are all different flowers in God's garden. Never, ever judge yourself by your accomplishments. Some people judge their self-worth by what they *get done*. Busy bees seem to be admired, right? But what if these busy bees sting? What good would that be? I would rather be around someone who was considered a little lazy, as long as they are nice.

Unfortunately anxiety and depression can sometimes come from what we think others think about us. If you can ever get the "hell with it" attitude, you will be a lot better off. A lot of people kill themselves, bending over backward, trying to please or impress other people. My sweet daddy instilled this attitude in me, and his mother, my grandmother used to tell me, "Tell them if they don't like the way it looks, look the other way!" Isn't that funny? But it is so true. Why are there so many women under the bondage of makeup? I used to be this way when I was a younger girl. You can't be seen without makeup on your face. I am happy to say that today I don't wear makeup at all, and I don't give a damn.

When you finally get to a point in life where you do your best, that's all you need. Unfortunately your best isn't good enough sometimes. That's when the judges move in. People will always move in quick to judge you. They do this because it makes them feel good about themselves. We know when we are being judged. Being judged can cause some of the most painful and intense anxiety on the market. It feels like quicksand being poured all over your body. You know it's really ironic, but as I am writing this portion, today, someone I love dearly has judged me and has been very critical of me. I *feel* the quicksand, and I feel the depression. I can't seem to shake it. Anxiety, depression, and mental deficiencies are things that are never completely conquered, just a work in progress, things that are *managed* from day to day, from month to month, from year to year. But for me that is ok. I have learned to accept it. Until you learn to accept it and live with it, you will never be happy, and happiness is something we all want, with mental illness or not.

If it takes you years to accept it, that's all right (because it did for me). Don't beat yourself up over it. In fact, never beat yourself up over anything because this can only increase your mental deficiencies. Learn that you are your best friend. Be good to yourself. Love yourself. While you're working on loving yourself, love others. Work on being kinder. Don't get me wrong—I'm not saying we are not kind people, but we can all work on being more kind and loving, starting with the people in your own family. Compliment others, work on lifting others up while you're lifting yourself up. If you find yourself alone and you *really* need someone to talk to, and there is nobody, then talk to Jesus. I play meditation music. It helps me with my anxiety. I like to get quiet and calm so that I can *think*. Just make sure it is positive thoughts you are thinking.

Control your mind; don't let your mind control you. As I write these passages, my main theme is love. Being kind to others, even when you don't feel like it, will benefit not only the one you're being kind to but also *you*. Kindness helps to ease anxiety and depression. Do you remember when you were little? You fell down and got a boo-boo, Mama would kiss it, and it was much better. Now you know good and well that Mama didn't have magic in that kiss, or did she? Of course, it was her kindness, covered in sugar. Just knowing that someone cared did all the good in the world. If you know someone who needs love, then give it. If you need love, then ask for it, in a kind way. Never demand it or make someone feel bad for not giving it in the first place.

One of my dear friends use to say, "There are many different flowers in God's garden." Some people are good at giving love and affection. Other people can seem more to themselves and standoffish. If you are depressed because of what someone else is or is not doing, then you are punishing yourself for nothing. Just try and focus on their good points. Because we are imperfect, it is easy to focus on the bad. When something is going bad, we home in on it. We think about it, and think about it. We worry, and worry, when there are so many good things to think about. Learn to control your mind. Make a conscience effort to *not* think about it. Say to yourself, "I choose not to think about [this or that] today."

As I write this, I confess that this is something that I am still working on. I have a sign on my wall that says, "Let go and let God." Do you know that this is one of the hardest things to do? I am one of the biggest worrywarts. I have four children and lots of grandchildren. It seems like there is always something going on. Something to worry about. But because I am imperfect, I can't help but be concerned about things. I can say that I am getting better at this technique. Worrying brings unwanted stress, and stress is not good for the body. Stress creates anxiety and is one of the mental deficiencies we talk about in this book. I don't know about you, but I hate stress, and I hate anxiety with all my heart. I like to stay calm, cool, and collected.

Let's talk about something else I hate that comes along with mental deficiencies: the stigma.

When someone is having or experiencing depression, bipolar disorder, or even anxiety, it is hard to stand up and say, "I need help." Why? Because of the way we are treated by society. If people didn't judge so harshly, or we were afraid of these people, we could not get more help. People who are having problems do not want to be judged. That is why people are so hush-hush about their problems.

Early in my life, there was a great family who lived across the street. I was childhood friends with their younger daughter. After growing up, my bipolar symptoms came out. There were times that I didn't know who I was or what I was doing. This scared them. Then one day they were all through with me. To this day I haven't seen or communicated with them. It's been about fourteen years, and I have been doing great with my bipolar disorder. I miss my friends to the point of crying about it from time to time. I hate even writing about my past experience because it brings me so much pain. That's what mental illness does. It brings you pain, whether it be past or present. I hate even saying "mental illness." I would rather say "mental deficiencies." There is something about the mind, when we're hurting mentally, and people tend to want to scatter, instead of being there for you like they should. Some people don't know how to handle it, or handle you, even if we are depressed or suffering from anxiety. Please don't rely on others to solve your problem unless they are professionals. Everyone has an opinion about what you should do, and they're usually all different.

This will mix you up even more. Remember, confusion is of the devil, and it will only make you sicker, not better. It may sound as if I am contradicting myself. I did tell you earlier to reach out for help to those who love you. What you need is for someone to *listen*, not tell you what to do. Finding someone who is like that may be hard. It seems like everyone and their uncle wants to tell you what to do or give you advice. You know God gave us two ears and *one* mouth. That means we should *listen* more and talk less. It may be a good idea just to say, "I need you to *listen*." Good luck!

I guess we've talked enough about other people. You can never change other people. The only one you can change is yourself. Changing yourself is good for anxiety and depression. Changing our way of thinking holds the key. I'm not saying there might not be some chemical imbalance in your brain. You know our brains are amazing. You have chemicals that affect the way you feel overall. I have bipolar disorder. That is a surefire chemical imbalance. I remember being a young woman and being in the middle of a manic state. With me my manic states would come three days in a row. Three days would go by without me being able to sleep at all. I would lay in bed and beg God for sleep, but sleep never came. By my third day of not sleeping, I would be like a drunk person, not knowing at all what I was doing. Half of the things I did I didn't remember. Then it was either off to jail or the mental hospital because of my erratic behavior. I have been hospitalized twenty-two times. I have only been to jail three times.

I am happy to say it has been fourteen years since I have been manic and couldn't sleep. I sleep like a baby now. Though I went through all of that, I never once blamed God. I know that though we may not understand, everything happens for a reason. That can be a hard one to understand and accept. But it is vital that we accept the things we cannot change, have the courage to change the things we can, and have the wisdom to know the difference.

Today I still experience anxiety. I have a nerve disorder called small nerve neuropathy. It brings a lot of pain to my body. I get really anxious when I'm in so much pain, yet I have to get things accomplished. Sometimes I have anxiety to the point of crying. My body hurts so bad, yet I have to push myself. There are times when I just cannot *go*. That is when I have to reschedule my appointment or activity. Jesus keeps telling me not to compare myself to others. My husband is my main competitor. He just goes and goes. He does so many things I should be doing, things that I'm not physically able to do. I feel guilty, even though I *know* I shouldn't. I have such a wonderful husband. He never complains.

How many times has Jesus told me not to compare myself to others? Everyone is different. If we are experiencing mental health issues, this takes away from us. Nobody knows how you feel but you. Feelings are real! They exist, and they can't be seen. You may look able bodied, but on the inside you may be dying. My sweet, belated daddy said to me, "You're so blessed. Why be depressed?" This is a very true statement but hard to put into action. Like I said earlier, being depressed is like being in quicksand. Your arms just can't move. Your body just can't move. If you not are able to *push* yourself, your spirit is down, way down. This is not what Jesus would have for us. When we are in this place, we have to hang on until we can get ourselves to a better place. Hanging on is the trick. If you have pushed yourself and gone to work, or done whatever you're supposed to do, then by all means *rest*. Lay your body down, curl up in a ball, do whatever makes you comfortable.

I remember one time when my boyfriend broke up with me. I was laying in my bed, and my friend came over and banged on my door. I just wanted her to go away, but she didn't. She knew I was depressed. She thought I should be up and at 'em. I did get up and let her in but then returned to my safe place. She went on and on about it, how I *needed* to get up. Please don't do this to anybody or let anybody do it to you. If your friend or loved one is experiencing depression, then just sit close to them. Pull up a chair or sit on the side of the bed. Show your love by touching gently. Keep your visits short and sweet.

I remember another time that I was depressed. I was in college. Boy, did my house get dirty! I did not have the will to clean up, not even behind myself. Have you ever heard of this? "The spirit is willing, but the flesh is weak!" That saying is in the Bible. My flesh was *so* weak. Well, during this time, a friend came over. I let him in because I just didn't care. He knew what was going on with me.

He immediately jumped in and started cleaning. That help was well appreciated because I knew he wasn't *judging* me.

Let's talk a little about that. Don't do it! "You never know what someone may be experiencing or feeling, because we are not in their body, or soul, and we just don't know. So don't judge. That's in the Bible too. I hope I'm not offending anyone who does not depend on God. That just happens to be what gets me through—God. Sometimes, not all the time, when you're experiencing anxiety or depression, you just have to get through. One day at a time, one hour at a time, one minute at a time. Hope is everything. Seeing that light at the end of the tunnel will be what helps pull you through to the other side. A side where you are no longer depressed, or no longer anxious to the point of not being able to function.

Anxiety and depression are not always extreme. I can be sitting in a chair, and one of my kids will catch me bouncing my leg up and down. Why? I had anxiety, and I didn't even know it. Having peace is a wonderful thing. When you have peace, you are calm. In the Bible it says, "Calm as a dove, but wise as a snake," which means just as it says: be calm, peaceful. Oh, what a wonderful experience.

Meditation always helps me. Remember, when you meditate, have good, positive thoughts. It does no good to meditate if you're just going to worry your way through it. If you catch yourself thinking negatively, take that thought and imagine flushing it down the toilet. Gone! Close your eyes and imagine yourself doing what you would be doing if you had all the money or time in the world. Would you be on vacation in the Bahamas? Would you be shopping? Would you be going to or eating at a fancy restaurant?

All of these things are positive. You may think it sounds silly, but not only are you drawing positive forces from the universe, but you are also replacing negative thoughts with positive thoughts. When you do this, you will also feel better overall. And while you are dreaming about more, more, more, don't forget to look around at what you already have and be grateful for it. If you are in the middle of a situation that brings you down, just look around. I'm not saying this will cure the problem, but it might help add a spoonful of positive thinking, kind of like medicine. While I was writing this insert, I, too, went through a little hell, but mine only lasted one day. I will tell you this: when you are in the middle of depression, it is really hard to count your blessings. I know; I get it.

We are imperfect humans, and we focus on the bad before the good. But at least try really hard to feel safe and warm in your own surroundings. There have been many times, especially in my younger days, when I was dealing with my bipolar disorder, that I did not feel safe and warm. In fact, I felt afraid and vulnerable. This is a hellish feeling, and it comes straight from the devil. The devil likes the negative experiences we feel. He plays with our brain and is the castrator of our mental disorders. Trust me; this is true. That's why we have to keep rebuking him away from us. Say it out loud: "Devil, I rebuke you in the name of Jesus." Fear is his biggest tool. So if you are experiencing anxiety or depression because you are afraid of the future, know that this is not what God wants you to feel.

We should keep our mind on the present. Jesus said in the Bible that we have enough cares in *today*. Tomorrow is not ours. Usually when we worry about tomorrow, it doesn't turn out the way we thought it would anyway. I know I repeat myself a lot in this book, but it's only the important things that might be said more than once. I repeat things like, "don't worry about your future" and "dream about good things." If you find yourself in the gutter, then take yourself out for a good meal. Order a cup of coffee afterward and enjoy yourself.

Also I believe in being nurtured when you're down. If you know someone who is experiencing anxiety or depression, then *baby* them. If you are the patient, then baby yourself. A little love goes a long way. Don't forget to touch. Hug someone. Rub someone's arm.

The human touch is a healing agent. Be *warm* and loving. If someone doesn't want to be touched, then just sit beside them. Just being there and being a good friend means everything, or having a good friend.

Let's talk about loneliness. When you're alone it's easier to experience feelings of depression. You have no one to talk to except Jesus. Instead of feeling lonely, try to take this time to think. Thinking is a great thing, and many great things have come from people who were alone. They have come up with ideas that brought forth inventions and great businesses. When you are alone, your creative juices can flow. I know that while I am writing this book, I am experiencing a lot of pain. Sometimes it seems so hard to live. I am only existing at times, so I know what pain is, whether it be physical or emotional.

But just remember that nothing ever stays the same—no, not even pain. Pain *will* eventually go away, I promise. The hard part may be getting through it, getting to the other side, and, yes, there is always another side. A light at the end of the tunnel. The trouble is some may not be able to see it. I know I experience my anxiety when I feel overwhelmed. I may be in a lot of pain, yet I have things I have to do. There have been so many appointments I have canceled because my body just won't go.

May I interrupt this passage by telling you that I have a baby rabbit? I went outside last night and took a baby rabbit away from my cat. I have him in a laundry basket in the laundry room. So far, he is still alive. What am I going to do with a rabbit? I think I will give him to my oldest daughter. She is good at raising wildlife. She has had squirrels. Well, it is sad to say the bunny died, but we tried, and that's all you can do in life—try. Try, try, and then try some more. Never give up. If you fall, then get back up. Sometimes stress and anxiety can cause you to lose your cool, you know, get angry. Have you ever just felt like you have so much piled on top of you? That's when I've lost my cool in the past. Feeling overwhelmed comes when you are going too fast. Slow down, be still! I've trained myself to take things one moment at a time. If tomorrow worries you or overwhelms you, then don't think about it. If there is something you need to do to prepare for tomorrow, then by all means go ahead and do it. Just take it slow and easy. You will have more peace that way. Peace in your mind keeps you healthy. You can eat all the fruits and veggies you want, but peace keeps your heart beating on a regular beat. Stress makes you sick, remember that.

I said earlier on that love is the theme of this book. It means as though we have been talking more about stress, depression, and anxiety.

During these times we desperately need love. Most people today don't realize how important love and affection are to humans' well-being. Remember Mama kissing the boo-boo? Well, didn't the boo-boo get better after that? Mental illness is the same as any other illness. It can rub off your overall well-being. But we do not want to be labeled as *sick*. I remember when bipolar disorder started with me. My daddy would always say that I was sick, and I hated it. I did not feel sick. In fact, I was in denial for a long time that anything was even wrong with me at all. One thing is for sure, if you are suffering from any kind of mental deficiencies, it is not your fault. Not your fault at all. Some people may act like it is your fault. I used to get accused of not taking my meds when I sure was. Being misunderstood comes frequently when you're sick. Everybody has your cure. Some say you should *get busy* to take your mind off things. You may not feel like getting busy. When you're not feeling good, you need to be left alone to decide for yourself what you feel like doing or don't feel like doing. Everyone is different. What might be right for one person may not be right for another. When I had depression, I wanted to sleep. Yes, sleep! I was sick, so I was entitled to rest. I had a friend once who came banging on my door. She didn't like it because I was in the bed.

Just remember, a true friend will leave you be. It's ok for them to sit on the side of your bed or sofa. It's ok for them to listen when you talk. What you don't need is someone trying to fix you. You, along with the help of time, will fix yourself.

If no one else is being kind to you, be kind to yourself. Go have a nice meal, or go buy that bottle of perfume you have been wanting. For the guys? Do something extra special. Just remember, whatever you're going through won't last forever. It's just temporary. Know this inside of yourself and make it your rule of thumb. I may not know everything, and I am far from perfect, but I do know this: love covers a multitude of pain. People need to stop going around judging one another and try a little love and kindness. A little love goes a long way. Love is a healing agent, along with time.

I have mentioned before that mental illness, or mental deficiencies, brings with it a lot of stigma. That is why so many people fail to speak up and get the help they need. If you ask me, I think the whole world needs help. These people who go around judging have their own issues to deal with.

I say the whole world needs help because we live in a world full of stress. Stress can contribute to our struggle, affecting our mind. That is why de-stressing is so important. Let me give credit where credit is due. The devil loves stress. Being stressed is the opposite of God's spirit, which is calm and cool. There are many times when I have to take my life minute by minute. I try really hard not to worry. Even though I try, I fail sometimes. Sometimes the circumstance is just too big. I forget to just let God have it.

Even though I preach about taking it minute by minute, I fall short sometimes. There will always be circumstances that push against our well-being. We have a fight with a loved one, lose someone in death, have financial problems. Oh my goodness. The list goes on and one. My sweet daddy taught me how to focus on breathing. He said as long as I am breathing, I am still alive. That is what we are all doing, trying to just survive. While we are surviving, we grasp for some happiness or pleasure along the way. That is why we have so many people who are all overweight. Eating is a given pleasure. In America we have turned everything into treats. Just yesterday my granddaughter wanted to go for ice cream. I had already made up my mind that I wasn't going to get anything. When I got there, the flavor of the day was Georgia Beach. There went my diet. I just had to have one scoop. Somehow I thought by eating this without the cone that I was being good.

You know, that's what it is all about—doing your best and letting others accept you just the way you are. No better, no worse, take me as I am. That is a dear, *true* friend. If you ever find a friend like that, hold on. That friend will cause you no anxiety, because you won't be stressed out trying to please them or to be what you think they want you to be instead of just being yourself. Don't be afraid to speak up. Tell someone exactly how you're feeling. Listen, when we are down, it may take the help of others to pull us up. Don't forget to keep telling yourself my sweet mama's words, "Sometimes you're up; sometimes you're down." That will remind you that there is an *up*, and you can have hope in that. Don't forget to focus on your breathing when you're breathing; you're still alive.

Now to change the subject a little. So much stress and anxiety comes from our financial standing. Yes, let's talk about money, the root of all evil, yet we all can't get enough of it. This is what people trust. This is what people put their faith in. God has been working with me in this area lately. He wants us to trust him instead of money. What? Did I just say something that offends people? How can we trust someone we can't see to provide for us? Anxiety comes from worry. We worry about *so* much, so many things. Yet everyone worries about not having enough money. Also, the more money we have, the more we spend, the more we get in debt. It's not really money we worry about; it's thinking of what will become of us if our money supply runs out. We are not trusting God, plain and simple! Taking it one day at a time helps calm the anxiety of worry, or anxiety that comes from worrying.

You know the saying, "Don't worry; be happy"? Well, it is a true statement. Happiness is obtainable. There is light at the end of the tunnel, and you have to march forward to it! Have hope. Learn to live in the moment instead of worrying about the future. Most of the time, the things that we fear never come to pass anyway. It turns out to be something else altogether.

There are many things that I will repeat in this book. The reason for repetition is that it is something very important, like living and worrying about *today* only.

Once upon a time, I didn't know about the importance of taking it slow and easy in your mind. Now that I know, it's the only thing that gets me through this chaotic life. Of course I use the words of the greatest teacher that ever lived, Jesus. He said to live one day at a time. He also said not to trust in money. He said God would take care of us. When you're anxious or depressed, don't you feel like you need someone to just take care of you? Lean on God. Trust him even though you can't see him. He is truly there with nothing but love for you. All you need is love. As I am writing this book, I can tell you that I love you. I love you because you are probably hurting. That's ok because hurting people heal and get better, and I pray this for you as well.

Remember what my daddy said: "Feelings come and feelings go, but what really matters is what you *know*." Know that you are a good person. Know that anxiety and depression don't last forever. Even bipolar disorder can be managed with the right medication. I'm living proof of that. *Know* that you are loved and needed in this world. You are special just because you are a child of God!

I know how mental deficiencies affect you. I am someone who has suffered a great deal because of it. Still, I have my moments. I grin and bear it until I get to a place of feeling better, and I always do.

Life is like a roller-coaster; sometimes you're up, sometimes you're down, and sometimes you're in the middle.

Dream, and dream big. Imagine yourself so blessed that you are a millionaire. Dream of all the things you would do and feel it as if it was real. I promise you that you will be blessed beyond your wildest dreams.

I'll tell you that there's something else that can cause anxiety and depression: *people pleasing*.

Just recently I have taken on a new attitude. It is the "I don't care" attitude. I have even started saying it out loud: "I don't care." You know the saying Elvis gave us: "I did it my way!" When you are constantly trying to please people, you can literally drive yourself nuts. Just know this: you can't please everybody all the time. I'm raising my eleven-year-old granddaughter. Everyone in my family has something to say about how I'm doing it. I've finally gotten to the point where *I don't care*! I'm doing it *my* way. I found out that this works! Someone started fussing at me. I quickly said, "I don't care," and that shut them up real fast. This took a lot of stress off me, and I was standing up for myself. I am not a pushover, and neither are you! Once we receive negative feedback from someone, it causes us to worry or fret. I'm not saying now that if someone gives loving advice that we can't receive that. If we see that, maybe we should change our way of thinking, but it has to be loving, and we have to receive it as truth. I'm talking about being fussed at or talked to like you have no sense at all.

You are a smart person, and you know what's right for you. If you are on drugs or drinking heavily, you might listen to a little fussing. Still, you are the captain of your own ship. You know what the right things are to do. You don't need people nagging you. Stop people pleasing.

Please yourself. Be good to yourself. Go to your favorite restaurant. Buy yourself a new outfit. Tell yourself over and over the good that you do and how good you are. Love yourself. Don't let anyone criticize you. If they do, just say, "I don't care!"

While you're doing all of this, don't forget to breathe. Your breath, and being aware of it, will focalize your mind. Once your mind is on your breathing, you won't be thinking about all your problems, or what you perceive as problems. Keep your mind on positive things. When your mind starts drifting to fears or negative thoughts, say out loud, "I rebuke you, Satan, in the name of Jesus." Control your thoughts—you can do it. Stop stressing. You are basically doing it to yourself. Rise above your situation and *live*. Live happily and choose to be happy.

Being happy doesn't mean you will go around skipping all the time. Being happy is a place where you are content, satisfied, and without emotional pain. Being in emotional pain is hell. I know firsthand what it feels like. When you feel this pain, just keep telling yourself that it won't last forever. You will rise above it. I can't say it enough: seek help. Finding a good doctor is your first step. Don't be afraid to take medicine. God put the medicine here to help us, not hurt us. Many times in the past, they would put me on a new medicine. I soon thereafter stopped taking it because I didn't like the way it made me feel. Give the meds a chance to adapt to your body. Give yourself time to adjust. If you slow down, then that's ok. Go with the flow. If you still aren't satisfied, discuss it with your doctor. Don't see having a doctor as a curse but rather know that you are special enough to have someone looking out for your best interest. Remember, there are people who care about you and your well-being, so seek these people out. I care about you, which is why I am writing this book. I want to help, even though I've never met you. You are special, and special people are greatly loved. Just imagine how much your creator loves you, more than you could ever imagine. So hold on tightly through your hard time mentally, until you get to a place of peace and pray, pray to God. He will guide you and help you.

There may be many things that I repeat in this book. Repetition is good because it helps you to remember. I repeat this: don't let your mind run ahead of you. That means take one day at a time. When we concern ourselves with the what if's in the future, we are setting ourselves up for failure. Nine times out of ten, it doesn't work out the way we worried about anyway. I'm just telling you what works for me. I take it slow and easy. I try not to let my mind—oh, that vicious mind—run away into the future. Taking it one day at a time works good for me. That's what our Lord Jesus told us to do. I suffer a lot with pain in my back. I have small nerve neuropathy. In other words my back is wacked out. Sometimes the pain in my back is so bad that all I can do is just lay down. I have to get *through* it, until I get to feeling better. That is what anxiety and depression are like. You just have to get through the valley until you get back up on the mountain. In all reality, that is what life is like for everyone, like my sweet mama says, "Sometimes you're up; sometimes you're down."

Lately, one of my friends has been suffering from depression. I have been calling her *every day* to check on her and ask her how she is feeling on the victor scale. She'll say about a four. To me four is below average. That's funny that I use a scale, one being at your worst and ten being at your best. As I am writing these words, I would say I am about a five, because I am in so much pain with my back. Sometimes my pain affects my feelings, and sometimes it doesn't. One thing is true: my feelings are always changing. Like my sweet daddy said, "Feelings come and feelings go, but what really matters is what you know." In other words he was saying to rely on your brain, not your feelings.

*Know* that you are blessed. Know that it could always be worse. *Know* that you will feel better in time. Nothing ever stays the same. Things are always changing. Sometimes you're up, and sometimes you're down, so make humor out of it. We can't be up all the time. Right now as I am writing this, I am about a five. Not too good, not too bad, somewhere right in the middle. I can remember the good times, and I can remember the bad times as well. Life is just like a roller-coaster ride, with all its twists and ups and downs. See life that way, and you will fare better all the way around. Just remember, God and Jesus know exactly what you're going through. God knows the number of hairs on your head. You are never, and I say never, alone with your feelings. They are just feelings; they are not *you*. But oh, don't those feelings feel like *you*, weighing you down? I am still trying to learn this valuable lesson from God. These feelings are not me, and they are not going to control me! I am going to control my thoughts and dream about winning the lottery.

My friend came over this morning. She is stressing over a particular situation. I gave her some good advice. I was telling her to take it one day at a time. That means keep your mind in today and don't let your mind run into tomorrow stressing and worrying. We can't control things that happen sometimes. The devil is always working, trying to disrupt us, but if we take the advice from the master Jesus Christ, we will not worry but give it to God and let it stay there. Letting it stay there is part of controlling your mind. If you keep worrying about something, you have taken it back out of God's hands. *Relax*. Everything will be all right.

Just yesterday I had to take my mom's cat to the vet. During our stay my back started hurting. I felt like it was going to break in two. I remembered what I have been trying to teach. I slowed down and started taking things one minute at a time, until I could get home and lay down. I tried not to focus on my pain but rather everything else around me.

When anxiety or depression, or any mental deficiency, has its ugly hands on us, we have to do the same thing. We have to put everything in our mind into slow motion and focus on all the blessings around us. This is hard to do sometimes, but if you can *control* your mind, you can get a handle on that racing mind. Calm it down, and in turn you will calm down.

I know y'all have heard me say before that I have a bad back. I have small nerve neuropathy, which means the nerves are wacko. There are times the pain is almost unbearable, just like with depression or anxiety. Sometimes you feel like you just can't make it through. Most of us don't have the luxury of taking time off from life. When you are suffering but have to keep going because your life demands it, it adds extra stress to you. When you're sick you need to rest, but sometimes that is hard to do. Just know that this is the time you have to take things real slow. Take one hour at a time. There are times I have to take it fifteen minutes at a time. I focus on Jesus and keep asking him to help me through.

I firmly believe that we as a society go too fast. It's progress after progress. I also believe it's this same society and progress that add to our stress level, which in turn leads to anxiety and depression. I know there can be other factors. Loss is something that we all have a problem with. If we could only see these losses as divine, we could dry up our eyes quicker. Those who die, I believe, go on to inherit great things and knowledge. We are the ones who mourn because we can no longer physically see or hear them. If we could only see behind the scenes, we wouldn't feel such pain.

I just recently dealt with two crises at one time. I used my techniques and, guess what, I made it through. Just like Mama says, "Sometimes you're up, and sometimes you're down." I always measure how I feel from one to ten. Right now as I am writing this passage, I am about a six.

When you're going through hell, draw close to Jesus and don't forget to breathe. You will get to a better time and place. Just be careful when you're down and don't take it out on others. Be kind to others, even if you have to fake it. Have you ever heard the expression "fake it till it's real"?

As I am writing this passage, I am down. My back is hurting so bad. This causes me anxiety. I will remember to breathe and try and keep my mind on my blessings and *positive* things. I want to be so full of Christ that if a mosquito bites me, it flies away singing, "There is power in the blood." Wasn't that funny? That is written on one of my coffee mugs that my dear, sweet daughter gave to me.

I have to be honest with y'all. These things that I write about, and the advice that I give you, are things I have to work on myself, day to day. Life is not easy all the time. I go through difficulties myself, and I try to apply my own advice. I have to remember to take it slow and easy, to take things one day at a time, sometimes one hour at a time. Even as we speak, I feel overwhelmed. So many things are going on in my life at one time. I can't tell you how important it is to your mental health to be, or get still, and *meditate*. By meditating we are able to talk to Jesus, knowing that he is there listening and communicating back with us.

I also have already told you how important it is to get help, which means finding and having a good doctor. I repeat myself a lot in this book but only because it is important. I have been seeing the same doctor for almost thirty years now. I take medicine for bipolar disorder and anxiety. Both work beautifully for me. I had a lady tell me not too long ago that she has bipolar disorder as well. She told me that her life was a train wreck because she did not have a doctor, nor was she taking any medication. Even if you do not have insurance, there are always programs out there to help the helpless. When I say *helpless*, that is not intended to belittle anyone who is without insurance. Helpless means you need help. Don't put it off. Do everything possible to live a good life. You have to be good to yourself and take care of yourself. You cannot do this alone. No one is meant to be an island. We need one another, and anyone with mental health issues needs a doctor.

My dear readers, since I wrote my last passages, I got sick with pneumonia. I felt like I was dying. I didn't want to die, but I really didn't know if I was going to make it. But I am back, still sick but not sick enough to where I can't write. What were we talking about? We were talking about mental deficiencies. If you ask me, I think the whole world has some type of mental deficiencies. Seems like the stress of this world causes all of us to need some sort of counseling. If you think you don't need counseling, think again. No one has it *all* together. If they think they do, just ask one of their family members, and they can tell you something that isn't so *all* together. And if you do have problems like me—bipolar disorder, anxiety, or depression—my dear, sweet reader, please don't feel bad about yourself, because I'm sure you have many good and righteous qualities.

The Bible says if you have faith as small as a mustard seed, then you will be saved. I always said, "Saved from what?" because I do not believe in a fiery hell where God sends bad people. We wouldn't wish that on our worst enemy, now would we? My goodness, that can give a person anxiety, just worrying about your future, both physical and spiritual. Don't worry; be happy. I know that is easier said than done. I just know that when we are mentally challenged, we need help. Whether we get that help from loved ones or from a total stranger, we cannot go it alone; no one is an island.

I am just quitting smoking. I know I need all the support I can get because it's not easy. My addiction to cigarettes is about to run me crazy, but I won't put another cigarette in my mouth. It is over. I am experiencing a lot of anxiety, so I will put my own advice to work and take this hour by hour. I will try not to work so hard, try to relax, and let Jesus take over. I will pour myself a hot cup of coffee, thank Jesus for it, and begin my day. I have some anxiety—no, I have quite a bit—but I can handle this one fifteen minutes at a time. I feel like I'm going to lose my mind.

Right now I am taking things five minutes at a time. It helps to write, so thank you, my dear readers, for sharing my stress with me. Stress is one of our biggest enemies. When you quit smoking, it is stressful, at least it is for me. But we won't think about that. I'm going to lay down for a while, listen to my mediation music, and dream about winning the lottery. Replace good thoughts with the fact that I can't have a cigarette. My chest is so tight and hurts, yet I want a cigarette. Now you know this is an addiction. I don't have to share all of this personal information with you, my sweet readers, but I am real, with nothing to hide. This is me, and maybe some of you can relate, or at least watch me go through anxiety and depression. I have already cried because I know I'll never see another cigarette again, which tells me I have an emotional attachment to cigarettes. I always said they were my best friend. So now I'm going to have to implement a little of my own techniques.

It's 3:50 a.m. I slept pretty good last night, so that's good. I'm not even thinking about a cig this morning, so that's good. Instead I'm thinking about all you wonderful people, friends, wishing I could be there with each and every one of you. I will say a prayer that for everyone who reads this book he blessed beyond all understanding.

Well, my friends, a couple of weeks have gone by since I wrote anything. Since then I have been in the hospital with pneumonia. I am home now. I am weak, but I am slowly getting better. I tell you I felt like I was going to die. I was not ready to die. I am only fifty-six years old. I have a lot of life left in me still. Now my mind is foggy but not too foggy to write. I guess you could say that I have anxiety. I will take things one hour at a time today. How I wish I could see my readers. We could all talk about our experiences together. I think being together and having support are very important. I have recently quit smoking. My son told me how very, very proud of me he was. Just that extra *very* helps me keep moving forward. If you take a step, say it's to go to the doctor, then you should be commended. Every step you take in managing your mental health is important. Be good to yourself, and take care of yourself. Nurture yourself. Eat a can of chicken noodle soup. You deserve it!

I've been out of the hospital for a week, and I feel like a baby. I am on oxygen because of my lungs. I am having a hard time because my anxiety is so high from wanting to smoke, but I'm finished with smoking, no more for me. I am trying to deal with my anxiety. As I continue to write, my anxiety is very high. Yes, I take medication for my anxiety, but my stress is still there. I have had a hard time finding Jesus even though I know he is there, helping me through. I remember my sweet daddy's words: "Feelings come and feelings go. What really matters is what you know." I *know* I will not smoke another cigarette. I *know* that smoking is detrimental to my lungs. I *know* I am getting healthy, my dear readers. I *know* you are going through this with me, just like I will be going through it with you when you read this book. I pray for all of you. Just imagine me sitting beside you on your bed. I will be there, coaxing you through the hard times as you make it through on your way to a better time. Just imagine that you can only go up when you are down, that is the only way to go—up, better. I am having a very hard time mentally without the cigarettes. I am going through depression now as I write. So, dear readers, I am just like you. I have my ups and downs. Right now I am down, or at least it feels that way.

I take out my Bible and read some. Then in the middle of my Bible I read a passage that says, "Living in the past is the only prison that will prevent you from soaring into an abundant future." I realize that I have been living in the past. I used to smoke, and people in my family said this or that about me. All of these things are in the past. I realize that I have to break free from my past. So many times we live in our past with regrets. If we don't do that, we live in our future with fear. Living in the now is what God wants us to do. We can eliminate a lot of our anxiety just by the way we think and what we think of or about. I have told all of you that I am quitting smoking, and my thinking has a big role in that. If I tell myself that it's ok to smoke, then I will. Oh my God, I would disappoint so many people if I went back to it after a month of smoke-free living.

Let's talk a little about self-punishment. I know this may sound crazy to you, but a lot of us love to punish ourselves. To some pain feels good. We love to think of negative things about ourselves or our situation that bring us fear or pain. Maybe you have been abused, and this is a familiar place. Being in pain by thinking negatively is a way of self-punishment. I know this is true because I have done it to myself. I would think about something that really hurt, and God would speak: Why are you hurting yourself? Then I would know. If you are puzzled when I say that God would speak to me, don't be. God speaks to all of us. We just have to learn to hear him. I would imagine I only hear about five things of what he says to me. You must be very still and quiet to hear him. Our brains are filters. We receive thoughts and then process them out. Negative things affect us negatively, and positive things affect us positively. And then we have our own thoughts. Yes, some are negative and some are positive.

How do you endure when the negative things take over? *Endurance* is a very important word when you're dealing with mental deficiencies. We have to, we must endure when the feelings are hard. When the times get really hard, we *must* endure. The Bible says that he that *endures* to the end will be saved. Hanging on is the key. When you are trying to *hang on*, you need to concentrate really hard. Concentrate on your breathing and keep your mind in the *now*.

My dear friends, I am about to close for now. Before I end, I would like to leave you with a few truths. First of all Jesus loves you very, very much. If you are suffering, just call out for that name: Jesus, Jesus, Jesus. He does not want you to suffer. He will help you to just give it a try. What do you have to lose? Nothing. Nothing at all. I will be praying for all my readers.

www.ingramcontent.com/pod-product-compliance
Lightning Source LLC
LaVergne TN
LVHW041542070526
838199LV00046B/1795